Metabolic Diet

A Beginner's 4 Week Step-by-Step Guide To Increasing Metabolism For Weight Loss: Includes Recipes and a 7-Day Meal Plan

mf

copyright © 2019 Bruce Ackerberg

All rights reserved No part of this book may be reproduced, or stored in a retrieval system, or transmitted in any form or by any means, electronic, mechanical, photocopying, recording, or otherwise, without express written permission of the publisher.

Disclaimer

By reading this disclaimer, you are accepting the terms of the disclaimer in full. If you disagree with this disclaimer, please do not read the guide.

All of the content within this guide is provided for informational and educational purposes only, and should not be accepted as independent medical or other professional advice. The author is not a doctor, physician, nurse, mental health provider, or registered nutritionist/dietician. Therefore, using and reading this guide does not establish any form of a physician-patient relationship.

Always consult with a physician or another qualified health provider with any issues or questions you might have regarding any sort of medical condition. Do not ever disregard any qualified professional medical advice or delay seeking that advice because of anything you have read in this guide. The information in this guide is not intended to be any sort of medical advice and should not be used in lieu of any medical advice by a licensed and qualified medical professional.

The information in this guide has been compiled from a variety of known sources. However, the author cannot attest to or guarantee the accuracy of each source and thus should not be held liable for any errors or omissions.

You acknowledge that the publisher of this guide will not be held liable for any loss or damage of any kind incurred as a result of this guide or the reliance on any information provided within this guide. You acknowledge and agree that you assume all risk and responsibility for any action you undertake in response to the information in this guide.

Using this guide does not guarantee any particular result (e.g., weight loss or a cure). By reading this guide, you acknowledge that there are no guarantees to any specific outcome or results you can expect.

All product names, diet plans, or names used in this guide are for identification purposes only and are the property of their respective owners. The use of these names does not imply endorsement. All other trademarks cited herein are the property of their respective owners.

Where applicable, this guide is not intended to be a substitute for the original work of this diet plan and is, at most, a supplement to the original work for this diet plan and never a direct substitute. This guide is a personal expression of the facts of that diet plan.

Where applicable, persons shown in the cover images are stock photography models and the publisher has obtained the rights to use the images through license agreements with third-party stock image companies.

Table of Contents

Introduction — 7
What Is a Metabolic Diet Good For? — 10
   Symptoms of gaining weight — 10
   Causes of Gaining Weight — 14
   Medical Treatments for Gaining Weight — 18
   Lifestyle Changes for Gaining Weight — 20
Metabolic Diet — 24
   Principles of Metabolic Diet — 24
   Benefits of a Metabolic Diet — 26
   Disadvantages of the Metabolic Diet — 28
   5-Step Guide on Getting Started the Metabolic Diet — 31
The Three Phases of the Metabolic Diet — 34
   Phase 1: The Reset Phase — 34
   Phase 2: The Metabolic Phase — 35
   Phase 3: The Lifestyle Phase — 35
Week 1: Learning What to Eat and What to Avoid — 37
   Phase 1 — 37
   Phase 2 — 40
   Phase 3 — 43
Week 2: Preparing Your Food the Right Way — 46
Week 3: Creating Your Meal Plan — 49
Week 4: Sustaining a Fast Metabolism through Healthy Lifestyle Habits — 52
   Eat natural, whole foods. — 52
   Follow a strategic fitness plan. — 53
   Eat within 30 minutes of waking up. — 53
   Try out new dishes, and incorporate new products into your weekly meal plans. — 54
   Stop thinking about calorie counts. — 54

Indulge yourself by eating your favorite food now and then.	55
Recipes	**56**
Mushroom Chicken Mix	57
Barley and Chicken Soup	60
New York Steak and Steamed Broccoli	62
Metabolic Boosting Smoothie	63
Butternut Squash Salad	64
Asparagus Farro Risotto	66
Barbecue Chicken Salad	68
Miso Beef Noodle Soup	70
Conclusion	**72**
References and Helpful Links	**74**

Introduction

Welcome to the ultimate guide to metabolic diets!

Congratulations on taking the first step towards a healthier lifestyle. Whether you're looking to shed a few extra pounds, increase your energy levels, or simply improve your overall well-being, the metabolic diet may be just what you need. In this guide, you'll learn everything you need to know about the metabolic diet, including its benefits, how it works, and how to get started.

First things first, what is a metabolic diet? Essentially, it's a way of eating that focuses on speeding up your metabolism. Your metabolism is the process by which your body converts food into energy. The faster your metabolism, the more calories you'll burn throughout the day. This can lead to significant weight loss, as your body uses its fat stores for energy instead of storing them for later.

So, how does it work? The metabolic diet is all about eating the right balance of macronutrients (carbohydrates, protein, and fat) to keep your body in a state of ketosis. Ketosis is a metabolic state in which your body uses fat for energy instead of carbohydrates. By keeping your carbohydrate intake low and increasing your fat intake, your body will enter this state of ketosis and start burning fat for energy.

Of course, like any diet, there are some foods you should avoid on a metabolic diet. These include processed foods, sugary drinks, and high-carbohydrate foods such as pasta and bread. Instead, you'll be focusing on whole, nutrient-dense foods such as lean protein, healthy fats, and low-carbohydrate vegetables.

But don't worry; a metabolic diet doesn't mean you have to give up all your favorite foods. There are plenty of delicious recipes and meal plans available that will keep you satisfied and on track. And, because a metabolic diet is all about balance, you can still enjoy the occasional treat without throwing your progress off track.

In this guide, we will talk about the following:

- What is a metabolic diet guide good for?
- Symptoms of gaining weight
- Causes of Gaining Weight
- Lifestyle Changes for Gaining Weight
- Medical Treatments for Gaining Weight
- Principles of a Metabolic Diet
- Benefits and Disadvantages of a Metabolic Diet
- 3 Phases of a Metabolic Guide
- Sample recipes of kimchi dishes

So, why should you consider a metabolic diet? For starters, it's a proven way to lose weight and improve your overall health. It can also be a great option for those with type 2 diabetes, as it can help improve insulin sensitivity and reduce blood sugar levels. And, because a metabolic diet is all about balance and nutrition, it can be a sustainable way of eating for the long term.

What Is a Metabolic Diet Good For?

Your metabolism is primarily responsible for how well your body allocates and uses up the energy it gets from the food and drinks you have consumed. The great thing about it is that metabolism can be directly influenced by your diet, your physical activities, and the quality of your lifestyle, in general. Therefore, to burn up the stored fats in your body and convert them into more energy to develop a leaner body, you have to commit yourself to a diet that can effectively speed up your metabolism.

As its name suggests, the metabolic diet is centered around these principles of weight loss. It encourages its supporters to eat highly nutritious foods and engage in regular exercise routines.

Symptoms of gaining weight

It is important to understand the different symptoms of weight gain or obesity before committing to a metabolic diet plan.

This will help you determine if your body needs the intervention of a metabolic diet.

Increased Body Fat

When a person gains weight, the excess fat can get distributed to various parts of the body, causing specific symptoms. The abdomen, hips, and buttocks are common areas where fat accumulation is noticeable. Fat accumulation in the abdomen can lead to a higher risk of developing health issues such as type-2 diabetes, heart disease, and stroke.

Gaining weight can also result in lower back pain, joint pain, and reduced mobility. Moreover, excessive body fat can affect hormone levels, causing adverse effects on the reproductive system.

Changes in clothing size

As an individual gains weight, clothing sizes may become a pressing issue. Tight or ill-fitting garments become a common occurrence, causing discomfort and dissatisfaction. Through weight gain, an increase in body fat leads to larger dimensions, resulting in a need for larger clothing sizes to accommodate this change. It is important to recognize that changes in clothing size, although an inconvenience, are a natural response to fluctuations in body weight and body shape.

Difficulty in physical activities

Gaining weight can significantly affect an individual's physical performance, making even the simplest of activities more challenging. Excessive weight gain can lead to difficulty climbing stairs, causing fatigue, shortness of breath, and body pain. It can also impact walking abilities, leading to slower walking speeds and increased chances of falls.

Furthermore, exercising becomes more challenging as excess weight puts pressure on the joints, making them more susceptible to injury. It's essential to maintain a healthy weight to avoid difficulties in these physical activities, thus promoting overall physical well-being.

Decreased energy levels

One of the most prominent symptoms associated with weight gain is decreased energy levels. This happens because the body has to work harder to carry the extra weight, thereby leading to fatigue and lethargy. Additionally, carrying extra weight puts pressure on the joints, making movement challenging and uncomfortable.

Such difficulties in performing daily tasks and remaining active can lead to a sedentary lifestyle, which, in turn, can exacerbate the effects of weight gain. Therefore, maintaining a healthy weight is crucial to ensuring a high energy level and overall physical fitness.

Joint pain

Gaining weight is a common symptom that can cause increased pressure on joints, leading to joint pain and discomfort. According to studies, for every pound of excess weight, there is four times the amount of pressure on the knees. Similarly, the hips are also impacted, with additional weight exacerbating joint pain and arthritis.

Furthermore, weight gain can cause inflammation in the body, which can lead to further discomfort and swelling in the affected joints. Therefore, maintaining a healthy weight through regular exercise and a balanced diet can help alleviate joint pain and prevent further damage.

Poor self-esteem

When individuals with poor self-esteem gain weight, they may feel an increased sense of shame and embarrassment. This is often due to unrealistic body image expectations perpetuated by society. Moreover, external pressure from peers and loved ones can exacerbate these negative emotions.

Women, in particular, are often bombarded with messages that thinner bodies are more desirable and attractive. Such messaging can be difficult to ignore and can contribute to feelings of self-hatred and low self-worth.

Sleep apnea

Weight gain is a significant risk factor for developing sleep apnea, a sleep disorder characterized by pauses in breathing during sleep. The extra weight around the neck and throat area can put pressure on the airways, causing them to narrow or even collapse completely.

This can lead to snoring, gasping, and difficulty breathing, which disrupts sleep quality and can cause other health problems such as high blood pressure, heart disease, and stroke. Losing weight through diet and exercise can help reduce the risk of developing sleep apnea and improve overall health.

If you are experiencing any of these symptoms, it's important to consult with a physician to determine the cause and create an effective treatment plan. A metabolic diet can be one way to decrease your weight, but it should always be done in consultation with a doctor.

Causes of Gaining Weight

There are several factors that can contribute to weight gain, such as overeating, a sedentary lifestyle, genetics, and family history, medications, medical conditions, poor sleep habits, and stress.

Overeating

Overeating is a common cause of weight gain because one consumes more calories than their body requires. The body stores extra energy in the form of fat, leading to increased weight gain over time. This can be attributed to factors such as unhealthy food choices, portion sizes, and a lack of physical activity.

Consuming high-calorie foods that are low in nutrients can also contribute to overeating, as the body doesn't feel satiated. Furthermore, eating at irregular intervals and skipping meals can alter metabolism and trigger overeating. Thus, making healthy food choices and engaging in physical activity can help prevent overeating and maintain a healthy weight.

Sedentary lifestyle

A sedentary lifestyle, characterized by a lack of physical activity, has been identified as a major cause of weight gain. This is because a decrease in energy expenditure can lead to an imbalance between calories consumed and calories burned, increasing body weight.

Furthermore, a sedentary lifestyle is associated with multiple health problems, such as heart disease, diabetes, and certain cancers. To combat the negative effects of a sedentary lifestyle, it is recommended to engage in regular physical activity, which can increase energy expenditure and promote weight loss.

Genetics and family history

It is not only genetics but family history as well that can determine one's propensity to gain weight. A study published in the New England Journal of Medicine shows that if both parents are overweight, their offspring have a 75% chance of becoming overweight themselves.

Moreover, research points towards hormonal imbalances and structural differences in the hypothalamus as weight-related factors controlled by genetics. Therefore, it is crucial to address these genetic predispositions along with lifestyle choices to prevent excess weight gain.

Medications

Certain medications, such as steroids or antidepressants, can cause weight gain. Antidepressants, specifically selective serotonin reuptake inhibitors (SSRIs), are notorious for causing weight gain due to their effect on metabolism and appetite. Steroids, on the other hand, increase hunger and cause fluid retention, resulting in weight gain.

It is important to note that not everyone who takes these medications will experience weight gain, and there are ways to manage this side effect, including exercise and healthy eating habits. However, it is essential to always consult with a healthcare provider before making any changes to medication or lifestyle habits.

Medical conditions

Hypothyroidism, a condition where the thyroid gland doesn't produce enough hormones, slows down metabolism, and can lead to weight gain. Polycystic ovary syndrome (PCOS), a hormonal disorder common among women of reproductive age, can also cause weight gain.

This is partly due to insulin resistance, which impairs the body's ability to use insulin effectively and leads to high blood sugar levels. Both conditions require medical treatment and lifestyle changes to manage weight gain and maintain overall health.

Poor sleep habits

Lack of sleep or poor sleep quality can have serious implications for regulating hormones related to appetite and weight management. One study found that sleep restriction resulted in increased appetite and cravings for sugary, high-fat foods. In addition, sleep-deprived individuals often experience decreased levels of leptin (a hormone that helps control hunger) and increased levels of ghrelin (a hormone that stimulates appetite).

These hormonal changes, combined with an increase in overall calorie intake due to increased appetite, can lead to weight gain over time. It is therefore important to prioritize good sleep habits as part of a healthy lifestyle.

Stress

Chronic stress, if not managed properly, can have a significant impact on an individual's weight gain. Stress can trigger overeating, particularly high-calorie and unhealthy foods, as a coping mechanism for emotional distress. It can also reduce motivation for physical activity, leading to a sedentary lifestyle that further aggravates the risk of obesity.

Chronic stress increases cortisol levels, a hormone that promotes fat accumulation, particularly in the abdominal area. The physiological and behavioral responses to chronic stress contribute to weight gain, making it crucial to manage stress levels through self-care practices, therapy, and other stress-reducing activities.

You need to understand the factors that can influence weight gain to create an effective and sustainable diet plan. The metabolic diet works by focusing on these underlying causes and providing lifestyle strategies to address them.

Medical Treatments for Gaining Weight

While lifestyle changes are generally the first line of treatment for weight gain, in some cases, medical treatments may be necessary. Here are some medical treatments for weight gain:

Prescription medication

Prescription medications that aid in weight gain are often used to treat conditions such as malnutrition, eating disorders, and certain illnesses. These medications work by increasing appetite, promoting the absorption of nutrients, and stimulating muscle growth. Common medications used for weight gain include appetite stimulants, steroids, and insulin. However, it is important to note that these medications should only be taken under the guidance of a healthcare professional and should be accompanied by a healthy diet and regular exercise.

Bariatric surgery

This type of surgery may be recommended for people who have a high body mass index (BMI) or suffer from other obesity-associated health conditions. Bariatric surgery can help reduce the amount of food the stomach can hold, leading to weight loss.

Thyroid medication

Thyroid medication can help regulate hormone levels and aid in weight loss if an underactive thyroid gland (hypothyroidism) is the cause of weight gain.

Polycystic ovary syndrome (PCOS) medication

For women who experience weight gain due to PCOS, medications such as metformin can help regulate blood sugar levels and insulin resistance, which can aid in weight loss.

Insulin management

People with diabetes who gain weight due to insulin resistance may need to adjust their insulin levels and take medications such as GLP-1 receptor agonists, which can help regulate blood sugar levels and promote weight loss.

Medical treatments for weight gain should always be discussed with a healthcare professional and should be accompanied by healthy lifestyle changes for long-term success.

Lifestyle Changes for Gaining Weight

The metabolic diet focuses on lifestyle changes to promote weight gain. Here are some lifestyle strategies that can be used in conjunction with the metabolic diet:

Balanced diet

Individuals who aim to gain weight have to make lifestyle changes to achieve their goals. As with maintaining a healthy weight, it is still crucial to consume a balanced diet, but with a focus on increasing caloric intake. This can be achieved by incorporating protein and healthy fat sources, like avocados and nuts, into all meals throughout the day.

Incorporating strength-training exercises into a workout routine can also help build muscle mass and aid in weight gain. It's important to note that weight gain should occur gradually, with a focus on overall health and well-being rather than quick fixes or unhealthy habits.

Portion control

Incorporating portion control into one's eating habits is a simple and effective lifestyle change for those looking to gain weight healthily. By decreasing portion sizes and avoiding overeating, individuals can regulate their calorie intake and ensure that they are consuming the appropriate amount of nutrients for their bodies.

In addition, practicing portion control can prevent the negative effects that come with overindulging, such as discomfort, bloating, and weight gain. Implementing this lifestyle change also promotes mindful eating, allowing individuals to savor their food and appreciate the flavors and textures. Taking control of portion sizes is a smart and healthy approach to gaining weight and maintaining a balanced diet.

Regular exercise

In addition to regular exercise, several other lifestyle changes can aid in healthy weight gain. Consuming more calories than one burns through daily activity is crucial. Eating nutrient-dense foods like whole grains, lean proteins, and healthy fats can help with weight gain while still promoting overall health.

Additionally, increasing meal frequency and choosing high-calorie snacks like nuts or nut butter can also aid in weight gain. Finally, ensuring adequate sleep and stress management are important, as lack of sleep and high stress levels can negatively impact weight gain efforts.

Adequate sleep

Incorporating adequate sleep is one of the most effective lifestyle changes for individuals struggling with weight gain. Research shows that individuals who sleep for at least 7-8 hours per night are less likely to overeat due to hormone regulation.

Additionally, getting enough rest can improve metabolism and energy levels, making it easier to engage in physical activities that aid with weight loss. It's important to prioritize sleep and create a consistent sleep schedule to achieve these benefits.

By following these lifestyle changes and incorporating a balanced diet, regular physical activity, adequate sleep, and stress management into your daily routine, you can effectively manage weight gain and create a healthier lifestyle. The metabolic diet works by guiding you to make these lifestyle changes to reach or maintain your ideal body weight.

Metabolic Diet

The metabolic diet is a nutritional plan that focuses on optimizing the body's metabolism to promote weight loss and improve overall health. It works by incorporating foods that boost metabolism and aid in fat burning, while also reducing or eliminating foods that can slow down the metabolism or contribute to weight gain.

The metabolic diet is designed to help individuals achieve their weight loss goals, and improve their metabolic health. By emphasizing healthy, whole foods and avoiding processed and sugary foods, the metabolic diet can help individuals achieve sustainable weight loss and improve their overall well-being.

Principles of Metabolic Diet

Balanced Macronutrient Intake
The metabolic diet emphasizes eating a balanced amount of protein, carbohydrates, and healthy fats for optimal energy balance.

High in Protein

The diet promotes the intake of lean protein sources such as chicken, fish, and legumes that help to increase satiety and reduce cravings.

Low Glycemic Index

The diet encourages the consumption of low glycemic index foods like whole grains and non-starchy vegetables that help regulate blood sugar levels, lower insulin production, and promote sustained energy levels.

Hydration

Staying hydrated by drinking enough water is essential for the metabolic diet as it boosts metabolism and helps to flush out toxins.

Frequent Eating

Eating small frequent meals throughout the day helps keep blood sugar levels stable and prevents overeating.

Exercise

Regular exercise, especially strength training, and high-intensity interval training can help boost metabolism by building muscle mass and improving insulin sensitivity.

Elimination of Processed Foods

Avoiding processed foods is a key principle of the metabolic diet as they are often high in added sugars, unhealthy fats, and calories that can slow down the metabolism and contribute to weight gain.

Portion Control

Paying attention to portion sizes is important in the metabolic diet as it helps control calorie intake and promote satiety.

By following the principles of the metabolic diet, individuals can boost their metabolism, increase fat burning, and achieve sustainable weight loss while improving their overall health.

Benefits of a Metabolic Diet

Weight loss

The metabolic diet can help individuals lose weight by revving up their metabolism and promoting fat-burning, while also reducing calorie intake from processed and sugary foods.

Improved insulin sensitivity

The diet's emphasis on low-glycemic index foods and balanced macronutrient intake can help improve insulin sensitivity and blood sugar regulation, reducing the risk of diabetes.

Increased energy

By eating whole, nutrient-dense foods that provide a sustained source of energy, individuals may experience increased energy levels throughout the day.

Better digestion

The metabolic diet's focus on whole grains, fruits, and vegetables provides ample fiber, which can aid in digestion and promote bowel regularity

Reduced inflammation

The emphasis on anti-inflammatory foods can help reduce inflammation in the body and lower the risk of chronic diseases such as heart disease and cancer.

Improved cardiovascular health

The metabolic diet has been widely recognized for its beneficial effects on cardiovascular health. By reducing levels of harmful cholesterol in the blood, it helps prevent the formation of plaques in arteries, reducing the risk of heart attack and stroke. Additionally, it promotes healthy blood pressure levels, further reducing the risk of cardiovascular disease.

Improved mental health

The metabolic diet has been found to have a positive impact on mental health by providing essential nutrients that improve mood, focus, and cognitive functions. A balanced intake of proteins, healthy fats, and fiber promotes the production of neurotransmitters such as serotonin and dopamine that regulate mood and emotion.

Following the principles of a metabolic diet can help individuals achieve sustainable weight loss, and improve their overall health. Eating a balanced mix of protein, carbohydrates, and healthy fats in combination with regular exercise and adequate hydration can help fuel the body with essential nutrients while promoting fat-burning and increased energy levels.

Disadvantages of the Metabolic Diet

Restrictive

The disadvantage of the metabolic diet lies in its emphasis on whole, nutrient-dense foods, which may feel restrictive for individuals used to consuming processed or high-calorie foods. This may result in some feeling as though their food choices are limited, leading to potential boredom with meal options.

Additionally, the focus on low-carbohydrate intake may cause individuals to feel fatigued or lethargic in the initial stages of the diet, as the body adjusts to a new way of obtaining energy. It is important to consult with a healthcare professional before beginning any new dietary regimen.

Cost

While consuming whole, organic foods can offer numerous benefits for one's health, a common disadvantage is the higher cost of such diets compared to other more readily available options. In particular, it can be difficult for low-income households to budget and afford such choices. The extra expenses stem from numerous factors, including the higher cost of organic farming and the limited availability of such products.

Despite these challenges, consuming whole, organic foods provides a wealth of nutrients, lowers exposure to harmful chemicals, and can prevent various diseases in the long run. Hence, it is essential to make informed choices that promote optimal health, while also finding cost-effective ways to incorporate these foods into one's diet.

Time-consuming

Despite the numerous benefits of following a metabolic diet, some disadvantages must be considered. One such disadvantage is the time-consuming nature of preparing meals using whole, nutrient-dense foods. This is especially true for individuals who have a busy schedule or lack culinary skills. However, it is important to note that the long-term health benefits of a metabolic diet outweigh these disadvantages. By reducing the intake of processed and high-sugar foods, individuals can improve their overall health, reduce the risk of chronic diseases, and foster a healthy relationship with food.

Limited social opportunities

The restricted choices offered by the metabolic diet can indeed pose a challenge, hindering individuals from engaging in social activities with their non-dieting peers. The dietary protocol is rigid, emphasizing proteins and cutting down on carbohydrates, fiber, and sugar. Consequently, it becomes impossible to enjoy the same meals with friends or family, often leading to social isolation.

Furthermore, individuals on the metabolic diet are restricted from eating certain foods, which might interfere with their ability to consume the same meals as everyone else. As a result, adhering to such a dietary regimen may induce psychological distress, exacerbate social anxiety, and negatively impact overall social interaction.

Although there are disadvantages, the benefits will be worth your time and effort. Following the metabolic diet can help individuals achieve sustainable weight loss, improved insulin sensitivity, increased energy, better digestion, reduced inflammation, improved cardiovascular health, and improved mental health. With the right approach and dedication to making healthier lifestyle choices, you can reap the full benefits of this diet.

5-Step Guide on Getting Started the Metabolic Diet

Getting started on the metabolic diet can seem like a daunting task. By following these five steps, however, you can set yourself up for success and begin to reap the benefits of this dietary approach.

Step 1: Determine your daily calorie needs

To get started with the metabolic diet, the first step is to determine your daily calorie needs. This can be achieved through the use of an online calculator or with the assistance of a registered dietitian. Both options allow you to ascertain the number of calories required to support your daily activity level while pursuing your weight loss goals.

By obtaining this information, you can tailor your food and beverage intake to ensure that you consume the appropriate number of calories needed each day to see results. It is important to remember that this number will be unique to you and your specific needs, so working with a professional is highly encouraged.

Step 2: Eliminate processed foods and sugary drinks

After determining your calorie needs, the second step is to minimize your intake of processed foods and sugary drinks. These items contain little nutritional value and can interfere with weight loss goals. While this does not mean that you need to completely eliminate all processed foods from your diet, it is important to ensure that the majority of your meals are composed of whole, organic, nutrient-dense foods. Additionally, sugary drinks provide empty calories and can spike blood sugar levels, leading to a crash in energy later on.

Step 3: Choose a lean protein

The third step is to select a lean and high-quality protein source. This could be animal-based such as fish, chicken, or eggs, or plant-based proteins like tofu, beans, legumes, nuts, and seeds. Protein is essential for muscle growth and repair as well as providing sustained energy throughout the day. Although high-fat proteins such as fatty fish, red meat, and full-fat dairy are allowed in the metabolic diet, it is important to limit these sources to no more than once a week.

Step 4: Add more whole, nutrient-dense foods

The fourth step is to incorporate more nutrient-dense foods into your meals and snacks. These could include vegetables, fruits, nuts, seeds, whole grains, legumes, and healthy fats such as olive oil or avocado. Adding these items will not only provide essential vitamins and minerals but also help you feel fuller for longer due to their high fiber content. Additionally, these foods will provide sustained energy throughout the day while helping to curb cravings and unhealthy snacking habits.

Step 5: Stay hydrated and exercise regularly

Finally, the fifth and last step is to stay properly hydrated and to exercise regularly. Staying hydrated will help ensure that your body is functioning optimally while also helping you maintain your energy levels throughout the day. Additionally, exercising regularly can help you burn additional calories as well as improve mood and reduce stress levels. These two elements are essential for long-term success with the metabolic diet.

By following these five steps, you can set yourself up for success and begin to reap the benefits of the metabolic diet. With dedication and commitment, it is possible to reach your weight loss goals while also improving overall health and well-being. Start small and be consistent in order to achieve the best results.

The Three Phases of the Metabolic Diet

This diet is designed to help you lose weight while keeping your energy levels high. The metabolic diet is composed of three different phases, each with its unique objectives and guidelines. Here are the three phases of the metabolic diet, along with their descriptions:

Phase 1: The Reset Phase

This phase lasts for two weeks and is designed to help reset your metabolism. During this phase, you'll be eating high-protein foods, healthy fats, and low-carbohydrate vegetables.

The goal is to eliminate sugar and refined carbohydrates from your diet, allowing your body to enter a state of ketosis. You'll also be drinking plenty of water to help flush out toxins and speed up the weight-loss process.

Phase 2: The Metabolic Phase

In this phase, you'll be slowly reintroducing healthy carbohydrates into your diet to keep your metabolism burning at a high rate. This phase lasts up to six weeks, and the goal is to achieve a more balanced intake of macronutrients.

You'll be eating a balanced mix of protein, healthy fats, and complex carbohydrates. This phase is designed to help your body maintain weight loss while keeping your energy levels high.

Phase 3: The Lifestyle Phase

The final phase of the metabolic diet is all about maintaining your newfound health and wellness. In this phase, you'll be making long-term dietary changes that will help you sustain your weight loss and keep your metabolism burning at a high rate. This phase is all about maintaining a balanced diet, regular exercise, and staying committed to your health and wellness goals.

The metabolic diet is an effective way to lose weight and get your metabolism back on track. Each of the three phases has its unique objectives and guidelines to ensure a gradual, sustainable transition to a healthier lifestyle. By following the metabolic diet, you can achieve your weight loss goals while keeping your energy levels high and improving your overall health and wellness.

By following these dietary guidelines, you would be ensuring that your body is still getting all the important nutrients during the diet itself. You need to maintain a good balance of complex carbohydrates, lean protein, healthy fats, natural sugars, and salt to meet your fitness goals.

It should be noted that the dietary changes you have to make occur in phases because you do not have to change everything at once. By doing it in shifts, the affected organ systems would have enough time to rest and recover, thereby keeping your body healthy throughout the entire course of this diet.

Following the prescribed schedule for your diet and exercise routine is critical for your success in losing weight through this method. Once you have gone through all the phases within a given week, you may repeat the cycle week after week until you have attained your desired body weight.

Week 1: Learning What to Eat and What to Avoid

For the first week of your metabolic diet, you should gain mastery over the kinds of food that you should be eating, and which ones you should avoid at all costs. Given that each phase of this diet requires a different set of macronutrients, the following suggestions are categorized according to which phase they would go best in.

Phase 1

Foods to Eat

In Phase 1 of the metabolic diet, you'll be resetting your body's metabolism through two weeks of high protein, healthy fats, and low-carbohydrate vegetables. Here are the foods you should eat during this phase:

- ***Protein source:*** Lean meats such as chicken, turkey, and fish, as well as eggs and low-fat dairy products. These provide essential amino acids for your body to build and maintain muscle while supporting a healthy metabolism.

- *Healthy fats:* Nuts, seeds, avocado, and olive oil. These provide the necessary fatty acids and oils that your body needs to function while keeping you full and satisfied.
- *Vegetables:* Non-starchy vegetables such as kale, spinach, broccoli, asparagus, and cauliflower. These are high in fiber, vitamins, and minerals that support overall health and weight loss.
- *Berries:* Small servings of berries such as strawberries, blueberries, and raspberries provide antioxidants, micronutrients, and natural sugars.
- *Water:* Staying hydrated is essential during Phase 1. Drinking water helps flush out toxins and supports your metabolism.

While these foods may seem restrictive, there are plenty of delicious and nutritious recipes available that can be incorporated into your meal plan. Be sure to avoid sugar, refined carbohydrates, processed foods, and alcohol during Phase 1 of the metabolic diet to achieve maximum benefits.

Phase 1 of the metabolic diet is crucial for resetting your metabolism through a gradual transition to a high-protein, healthy fat, and low-carbohydrate vegetable diet. By incorporating the right foods into your meal plan, you can improve your overall health, support weight loss, and boost your metabolism.

What to Avoid

In Phase 1 of the metabolic diet, there are certain foods that you should avoid to achieve the maximum benefits of the diet. Here are the foods that you should avoid during Phase 1:

- ***Refined carbohydrates:*** These include white bread, pastries, cakes, and other processed foods that contain little to no nutrition and can cause unhealthy weight gain.
- ***Sugar:*** This includes any foods or drinks with high amounts of added sugar, such as sodas, energy drinks, and sweetened juices.
- ***Starchy vegetables:*** While non-starchy vegetables are encouraged during Phase 1, starchy vegetables like potatoes, peas, and corn should be avoided or limited.
- ***Alcohol:*** Alcohol consumption can hinder metabolic function by slowing down the metabolism, contributing to inflammation and dehydration, and adding unnecessary calories to your diet.

By avoiding these foods during Phase 1, your body is better able to reset and adjust to a higher protein, healthy fat, and low-carbohydrate vegetable diet. It is essential to stick to the recommended food list during this phase to achieve maximum benefits, including improved weight loss, energy levels, and overall health.

Phase 1 of the metabolic diet requires avoiding certain foods to promote a healthy and sustainable transition into the diet. By avoiding refined carbohydrates, sugar, starchy vegetables, and alcohol, you can help reset and boost your metabolism, support healthy weight loss, and improve your overall health.

Phase 2

What to Eat

In Phase 2 of the metabolic diet, you will be reintroducing healthy carbohydrates to your diet gradually. Here are the foods you should eat during this phase:

- *Protein sources:* Same as Phase 1, such as chicken, turkey, fish, eggs, and low-fat dairy products. These provide essential amino acids for your body, building and maintaining muscles, and supporting a healthy metabolism.
- *Healthy fats:* Nuts, seeds, avocado, and olive oil, provide the necessary fatty acids and oils needed to function while keeping you full and satisfied.
- *Vegetables:* Non-starchy and starchy vegetables such as broccoli, cauliflower, carrots, beets, and sweet potatoes. These provide the essential vitamins, antioxidants, and fiber needed for overall health and weight loss.
- *Fruits:* Limited amounts of sugar from fruits in your diet are allowed, such as berries, apples, and pears.

- ***Whole grains:*** Reintroduce whole grains such as quinoa, brown rice, and oats in small amounts.

Similar to Phase 1, it is recommended to increase water intake during Phase 2 to flush out toxins and support your metabolism.

Phase 2 of the metabolic diet focuses on incorporating healthy carbohydrates into your meal plan, while still maintaining a high protein and healthy fat diet. By gradually increasing your carbohydrate intake and sticking to healthy, nutrient-dense foods, you can continue to support your weight loss goals while increasing your energy levels.

What to Avoid

The Phase 2 Metabolic Diet Guide emphasizes a healthy, balanced diet to promote weight loss and improve overall health. Here are some of the foods to avoid in this diet:

- ***Processed foods:*** These foods tend to be high in calories, unhealthy fats, sugar, and salt. Processed foods can lead to weight gain and increase the risk of chronic health conditions.
- ***High-glycemic-index (GI) foods:*** Foods with a high glycemic index can cause a quick spike in blood sugar levels, which can lead to insulin resistance and weight gain. Examples of high-GI foods include sugary drinks, white bread, and pastries.

- ***Sugar and artificial sweeteners:*** Added sugar and artificial sweeteners are high in calories and can contribute to weight gain. They can also disrupt the body's ability to regulate blood sugar levels.
- ***Trans fats:*** Trans fats are unhealthy fats that occur in processed foods such as fried foods, baked goods, and margarine. Trans fats can lead to inflammation in the body and increase the risk of heart disease.
- ***Alcohol:*** Alcoholic drinks are high in calories and can contribute to weight gain. Regular alcohol consumption can also lead to an increased risk of liver disease, cancer, and other health problems.
- ***High-fat dairy products:*** High-fat dairy products, such as cheese and butter, are calorie-dense and can contribute to weight gain. Choosing low-fat dairy products can help reduce calorie intake.
- ***Fried foods:*** Fried foods are high in calories and unhealthy fats that can contribute to weight gain and increase the risk of heart disease.

By avoiding these foods and focusing on a diet rich in whole foods like fruits, vegetables, lean protein, and healthy fats, individuals can promote weight loss and improve their overall health.

Phase 3

What to Eat

The Phase 3 Metabolic Diet Guide emphasizes adopting a healthy, balanced diet to maintain weight loss and improve overall health. Here are some of the foods that are recommended to eat in this diet:

- *Whole grains:* Whole grains, such as brown rice, quinoa, and oats, are rich in fiber, which can aid in digestion and promote satiety. They are also low glycemic index foods and provide energy for the body.
- *Fruits and vegetables:* Fruits and vegetables are packed with vitamins, minerals, and antioxidants that can help reduce inflammation and promote overall health.
- *Lean protein:* Lean protein sources, such as chicken, fish, and legumes, can help promote muscle development and satiety, reducing hunger and aiding in weight maintenance.
- *Healthy fats:* Healthy fats, such as those found in avocados, nuts, and olive oil, can help reduce inflammation in the body, improve brain function, and promote satiety.
- *Low-fat dairy products:* Low-fat dairy products, such as skim milk and low-fat yogurt, are good sources of protein and calcium while being low in calories.

- *Water and other healthy beverages:* Adequate fluid intake and choosing healthy beverages such as green tea can help prevent dehydration and promote weight management.

By following a well-balanced diet that focuses on whole, healthy foods, individuals can maintain their weight loss and improve their overall health.

What to Avoid

While focusing on a well-balanced diet rich in nutrient-dense foods is recommended in the Phase 3 Metabolic Diet Guide, some foods should be limited or avoided. Here are some of them:

- *Processed foods:* Processed foods, such as fast food, snack cakes, and frozen meals, are often high in unhealthy fats, sugar, salt, and calories, which can contribute to weight gain and chronic health conditions.
- *Sugar and artificial sweeteners:* Added sugar and artificial sweeteners are high in calories, can contribute to weight gain, and can disrupt the body's regulation of blood sugar levels.
- *High-fat meats:* Fatty meats, such as bacon, sausage, and fatty beef, can be high in calories and unhealthy fats, which can contribute to weight gain and increase the risk of heart disease.

- ***White bread and pasta:*** Highly processed bread and pasta can have a high glycemic index, leading to a quick spike in blood sugar levels and contributing to insulin resistance and weight gain.
- ***Fried foods:*** Fried foods are often high in unhealthy fats and calories, which can contribute to weight gain and increase the risk of heart disease.
- ***Alcohol:*** Alcoholic drinks are high in calories and can contribute to weight gain. Regular alcohol consumption can also lead to an increased risk of liver disease, cancer, and other health problems.

By avoiding or limiting these foods and instead focusing on whole, nutrient-dense foods such as whole grains, fruits and vegetables, lean protein, healthy fats, and low-fat dairy, individuals can maintain their weight loss and improve their overall health.

In Phases 1-3, the Metabolic Diet Guide provides an effective way to achieve sustainable weight loss and improve overall health. By focusing on whole, nutrient-dense foods, limiting processed foods and sugar, and avoiding fried foods and alcohol, individuals can maintain their weight loss results and reduce their risk of developing chronic health conditions such as heart disease.

Week 2: Preparing Your Food the Right Way

Now that you know the types of food that you can eat, the next step of your journey is learning how to prepare them according to the standards of the Metabolic Diet. Even though you may have bought your food from a local and organic source, it may still contain components that can disrupt your fast metabolism.

To minimize this likelihood, here are some essential tips on how to properly prepare your food:

- Get rid of the visible fats and skin from meat, poultry, and seafood.
- Wash fruits and vegetables thoroughly using running water from the tap. Let them air-dry if you have enough time to do so.
- To eliminate traces of pesticide from your produce, peel off the skins from vegetables and fruits, whenever applicable.

- Remove the top portions of fruits, such as apples and oranges. Pesticides might have been absorbed through the stem area.
- Dispose of the outer layers of lettuce, cabbage, and other similar vegetables since they are exposed to potentially harmful elements from the environment.
- Do not fry meat, poultry, or seafood products. You may bake, grill, or broil them instead.
- If you choose to grill your food, make sure that you are cooking lean cuts only.
- Fattier cuts are more prone to burning, which also means that more carcinogens would build up in your food.
- Do not save up the juices that have dripped off from grilled meat, poultry, or seafood.
- Turn over your food only once during the cooking process, normally during the middle of the total cooking time. Doing so would prevent it from being burnt up, while still allowing it to gain an appealing golden brown color.
- In case you need something to cover your food while cooking it in the microwave, use an inverted ceramic or glass dish, or a chlorine-free paper towel instead of plastic covers.
- If you prefer decanting or transferring your food into dedicated containers, opt for glass containers rather than plastic ones.

- If you have to wrap your food before storing it away, make it a point to use only BPA-free wraps.

Make a habit out of these food preparation tips by observing and practicing them regularly. Remember to follow them as well when you recreate the recipes given in the latter section of this guide.

Week 3: Creating Your Meal Plan

At this point, you are well equipped with the knowledge of what food to include in your meal plan, as well as the techniques you need to prepare them correctly. Based on what you have learned so far, you can now create a meal plan that follows the dietary guidelines for each phase of the Metabolic Diet.

To demonstrate how you could go about this, here is a sample 7-day meal plan that showcases the points covered in the previous chapters of this guide. Observe the combination patterns so that you can apply them to your meal plan.

7-day meal plan

	AM (breakfast and snack)	Noon (lunch and snack)	PM (dinner)
Day 1	Berry Smoothie	Mushroom Chicken Mix	Halibut Skewers with Onions and Eggplant
	Unsalted Walnuts	Orange Slices	
Day 2	Burrito	Barley and	Chipotle Beef

		Chicken Soup Hot Tuna Sandwich	Vegetable Tacos
	Carrot Sticks and Hummus Dip	Sunflower Seeds	
Day 3	Spanish-Style Scrambled Egg Whites	New York Steak and Steamed Broccoli	Southwest Chicken Salad
	Blueberries	Black Beans and Tomato Salsa	
Day 4	Metabolic Boosting Smoothie	Lemon Garlic Shrimp with Grilled Vegetables	Butternut Squash Salad Grilled Pork Chop with Steamed Beans
	Morning Snack Unsalted Walnuts	Low-Fat Mozzarella Sticks	
Day 5	Parfait	Grilled Chicken Breast Steamed Spinach with Mushrooms and Garlic	Wild Pacific Salmon with Roasted Vegetable Asparagus Farro Risotto
	Dry-Roasted Almonds	Non-Fat Greek Yoghurt	
Day 6	Egg White Omelet with Tomato Slices	Pork Tenderloin with Mushroom Gravy Roasted Asparagus	Barbecue Chicken Salad Split Pea Soup
	Cucumber and Hummus Dip	Afternoon Snack Watermelon Slices	

Day 7	Oatmeal with Low-Fat Milk	Miso Beef Noodle Soup Vietnamese Spring Rolls	Grilled Tuna Lemon Braised Vegetables
	Raw Almonds	Mixed Berries	

Week 4: Sustaining a Fast Metabolism through Healthy Lifestyle Habits

Your metabolism is not a fixed aspect of your life. You have to learn how to optimize your daily habits to maintain the high metabolism rate that you have achieved for the past few weeks.

There is no one secret strategy that you may follow. Instead, you have to abide by these six guiding principles of a fast, but healthy metabolic rate. By doing so, you would be able to gradually take control of how much weight you will gain or lose.

Eat natural, whole foods.

You have learned during your first week the making of a proper high metabolic diet. Continue to create your succeeding meal plans following those rules to keep your metabolic rate up to where you want it to be.

Go for foods that have been grown organically. May it be fruits, vegetables, meat, or seafood, choose something that you can purchase locally to ensure the freshness of the food you are eating.

Avoid at all costs all processed foods, especially those that contain artificial sweeteners, preservatives, and colorings. Health experts have identified these man-made additives as highly disruptive of key metabolic processes within your body.

Follow a strategic fitness plan.

To keep up the rate of fat-burning activities inside your body, you should engage in a combination of cardio and strength exercises every week. If you do not, then your adrenals would have to break down your muscles for fuel instead, thereby ruining the progress you have made in building up your muscle tissues.

Remember to eat a small snack before starting your workout routine. This would further stimulate the positive effects of exercises on your body.

Eat within 30 minutes of waking up.

Forcing your body to operate without fuel would be counterintuitive to your weight loss initiatives. If you forgo eating your breakfast, the cortisol hormones from your adrenals would trigger your body to begin storing up more fat in preparation for the possibility of being starved for the rest of the day.

To prevent this from occurring, you must eat your breakfast as soon as you have woken up. You do not have to eat a heavy meal to start your day right. Many experts on metabolism recommend consuming small, but frequent meals throughout the day, rather than three big meals during breakfast, lunch, and dinner times only.

Try out new dishes, and incorporate new products into your weekly meal plans.

You might think that eating the same combination of foods every week would help you sustain a fast metabolism. However, studies show that sticking to the same meals regularly can lead to a metabolic plateau. When this happens, the body would begin stockpiling fats again, and the production of energy would gradually decrease.

You may keep yourself from reaching the metabolic plateau by learning new recipes, and including them in your weekly meal plans. You should also shop for different varieties of fresh produce and meat products every week.

Stop thinking about calorie counts.

Keep in mind that eating less can slow down the rate of your metabolism. A slow metabolism would lead to a build-up of unnecessary fats in your body.

Rather than restricting yourself by counting the calories in every food you eat, you should focus instead on the quality of food that you are going to eat. Go for highly nutritious, organically grown food products, since they may be consumed in great quantities without harming your body and negatively affecting your metabolism.

Indulge yourself by eating your favorite food now and then.

Completely avoiding the food that you enjoy eating is not a realistic and sustainable lifestyle strategy. Studies show that eating one's favorite food promotes the release of endorphins, and reduces the production of cortisol.

Therefore, you should not feel guilty about indulging yourself now and then with a slice of your favorite pie or drinking hot chocolate with tiny marshmallows in it. They do serve a purpose in keeping you healthy in the long run, and you may counteract their negative effects on your body by consuming healthy and natural food products for the majority of the time.

Recipes

For your reference, here are the recipes of some of the menu items given in the sample 7-day meal plan in Chapter 5 of this guide. Each of these recipes is guaranteed to be within the standards of the Metabolic Diet.

If you wish to increase the number of servings of a particular dish, simply adjust the quantities stated in the ingredient list accordingly. You may also alter the ingredients according to your personal preference, as long as it still follows the dietary requirements of the diet.

Mushroom Chicken Mix

Ingredients:

- 4 chicken thighs, bone-in and skin removed
- 8 oz. (around 3 cups) of baby Bella mushroom, sliced
- 4 oz. (around 1 ounce per slice) of nitrate-free turkey bacon, diced
- 4 cups fresh baby spinach
- 4 cups cauliflower rice, steamed
- 3/4 cup coconut milk
- 3 cloves garlic, minced
- 2 tbsp. extra-virgin olive oil, divided into two
- 2 tsp. Italian seasoning
- 5 sprigs of fresh thyme
- sea salt
- freshly ground black pepper

Instructions:

1. Preheat the oven to 375°F (191°C).
2. Place the bacon in an oven-proof skillet with 1 tablespoon of oil and a medium heat setting.
3. Fry bacon until it becomes crispy.
4. Transfer the bacon to a plate using a slotted spoon.
5. Leave the bacon oil in the skillet.
6. Add another tablespoon of oil to the skillet.
7. Increase the heat setting to medium-high.

8. Rub both sides of the chicken thighs with salt, pepper, and Italian seasoning.
9. Place the meaty side of the chicken thighs on the surface of the hot skillet.
10. Cook without flipping over the chicken thighs for around 7 minutes, or until the meaty sides have turned golden brown and can be easily removed from the pan.
11. Flip the chicken thighs to the other side.
12. Transfer the skillet to the preheated oven.
13. Bake for 13 minutes, or until the internal temperature of the chicken thighs has reached 160 0F (71 0C).
14. Transfer the chicken thighs to a plate.
15. Return the skillet to the stovetop.
16. Add the mushrooms to the skillet.
17. Cook in medium-high heat for 4 minutes, or until mushrooms have become golden brown and a bit soft. Stir only mid-way through this step.
18. Add the garlic to the skillet.
19. Sauté for about 30 seconds to 1 minute, or until it has become fragrant.
20. Add the coconut milk, thyme, and ¼ teaspoon of sea salt into the skillet.
21. Gradually bring to a boil, then reduce heat from medium-high to low.
22. Simmer for around 2 to 4 minutes, or until the sauce has been slightly reduced and the flavors have blended well.

23. Stir in the fried bacon.
24. Sprinkle it with salt and pepper, to taste.
25. Place back the chicken thighs into the skillet.
26. Coat all over each thigh with sauce.
27. Combine the steamed cauliflower rice and spinach.
28. Arrange the chicken, cauliflower rice, and spinach on serving plates.
29. Serve immediately.

Yield: 4 servings

Tip #1: For the cauliflower rice, you may either steam a 16-ounce bag of cauliflower or create your own by running a pound of fresh cauliflower into a food processor.

Tip #2: Exercise extra care when transferring the skillet from the oven. The handle will be very hot.

Barley and Chicken Soup

Ingredients:

- 4 cups vegetable broth
- 4 cups chicken broth
- 2-1/2 lb. chicken breast, cubed, bone and skin removed
- 2 cups butternut squash, peeled and cubed
- 2 cups yellow summer squash
- 2 cups cubed zucchini squash
- 1 cup white onion, diced
- 1 cup broccoli florets
- 8 oz. fresh mushrooms, chopped
- 1 cup barley
- 2 cups water
- 1 tbsp. garlic, minced
- 1 whole bay leaf
- 1/4 tsp. sea salt
- 1/4 tsp. ground black pepper

Instructions:

1. Pour the water, vegetable broth, and chicken broth in a large pot.
2. Add the chicken cubes, onion, garlic, bay leaf, salt, and black pepper.
3. Using medium-high heat, bring the contents of the pot to a boil.
4. Reduce the heat to low. Simmer for an hour.

5. Add the barley, broccoli, butternut squash, yellow summer squash, zucchini, and mushrooms into the pot.
6. Bring back to a boil.
7. Lower it to a simmer for about 60 to 120 minutes, or until vegetables have achieved your desired texture.
8. Transfer into a serving bowl immediately.

Yield: 8 to 10 servings

New York Steak and Steamed Broccoli

Ingredients:

- 6 oz. New York Strip Steak, excess fat removed
- 3 cups broccoli florets
- 1/2 tsp. garlic, minced
- 1/2 tsp. sea salt
- 1/8 tsp. ground black pepper*

Instructions:

1. Preheat the broiler and broiler pan.
2. Rub both sides of the steak with garlic, salt, and pepper.
3. Place the steak on the hot broiling pan.
4. Broil for 7 to 15 minutes or until the desired doneness has been achieved.
5. Steam broccoli in the microwave or stovetop using a bowl of 2-inch deep water.
6. Sprinkle it with salt and pepper to taste.
7. Transfer steak onto a plate.
8. Transfer steamed broccoli to the side of the steak or in a separate bowl.
9. Serve immediately.

*black pepper may be substituted with white pepper

Yield: 2 to 3 servings

Metabolic Boosting Smoothie

Ingredients:

- 6 oz. vanilla, non-fat Greek yogurt
- 1 cup strawberries, frozen
- 3/4 cup iced green tea
- 1/4 cup broccoli florets, stems removed
- 1/4 cup garbanzo beans or cannellini
- 1 tsp. flax meal
- 1/4 tsp. ground cinnamon
- 8 pcs. almonds

Instructions:

1. Put all ingredients into a blender.
2. Blend until the texture has become smooth.
3. Transfer into a glass or preferred container.
4. Sprinkle ground cinnamon on top.
5. Serve immediately.

Yield: 1 to 2 servings

Butternut Squash Salad

Ingredients:

- 1 butternut squash, medium-sized, peeled and cubed
- 5 cups kale, chopped
- 2 cups farro, raw
- 1/2 cup shallot, diced
- 2-1/2 extra-virgin olive oil
- 1 tbsp. grapeseed oil
- 1 tsp. sea salt
- 1/2 tsp. ground black pepper
- 1 lemon, juiced
- 5 cups water or stock

Instructions:

1. Preheat oven to 400℉ with the oven rack positioned in the middle.
2. Toss the butternut squash in 1-1/2 tbsp. olive oil, salt, and pepper.
3. Roast butternut squash for 15 to 20 minutes.
4. Cook 2 cups of farro with 5 cups of water or stock and a tablespoon of olive oil in a rice cooker.
5. Heat the grapeseed oil in a pan using the medium setting of the stove.
6. Add shallots when bubbles start forming.
7. Cook for 2 minutes.
8. Add the kale to the pan along with the lemon juice.

9. Once the kale has turned soft, add the cooked farro and butternut squash.
10. Transfer into a bowl.
11. Serve.

Yield: 3 to 4 servings

Tip: Use the setting for cooking brown rice in your rice cooker, if available.

Asparagus Farro Risotto

Ingredients:

- 4 cups low-sodium vegetable broth
- 2 cups farro
- 1-1/4 cup dry white wine
- 1 cup asparagus, cut into 1-inch pieces
- 1 cup pea, frozen
- 2 cloves garlic, minced
- 1 shallot, diced
- 2 tbsp. extra-virgin olive oil
- 2 tbsp. butter, regular
- 2 tbsp. butter, unsalted
- 1/3 cup parmesan cheese, grated
- salt
- cracked black pepper

Instructions:

1. Blanch or roast the asparagus.
2. Using a heavy saucepan, heat the olive oil and butter together.
3. Add the shallots. Cook until the shallots have become soft and transparent.
4. Add the farro and garlic. Stir the pan until the farro and garlic have been coated by the oil.
5. Cook for a few minutes until farro and garlic has been toasted.

6. Pour the white wine.
7. Using medium heat, cook while stirring often until the wine has been completely absorbed by the other ingredients.
8. Add the broth, one cup at a time.
9. Stir the farro as you continue adding cups of broth.
10. Cook the farro for another 25 to 30 minutes, or until the texture has become al dente.
11. Add the peas and asparagus. Stir well.
12. Remove the mixture from the stove.
13. Stir in more butter and grated parmesan cheese.
14. Transfer into individual bowls with a side of grated parmesan cheese, and cracked black pepper.

Yield: 4 servings

Barbecue Chicken Salad

Ingredients:

- 2 grilled chicken breasts, sliced
- 1/2 cup pre-made barbecue sauce
- 1-1/2 lbs. asparagus, cut into 1-inch pieces
- 1 cup French lentils OR green lentils, well rinsed
- 1 chipotle chili in adobo sauce
- 1 tablespoon adobo sauce
- 4 stalks of celery, chopped
- 2-1/2 cups water
- 1/4 cup walnuts, lightly toasted and chopped

Instructions:

1. Put the lentils, chipotle chili, adobo sauce, and water in a rice cooker.
2. Press the cook button.
3. Add the asparagus as soon as the rice cooker stops.
4. Cover the rice cooker once more to steam the contents for 5 minutes.
5. Transfer the lentil mixture from the rice cooker into a bowl without cover.
6. Place the grilled chicken slices in another medium-sized bowl.
7. Add the celery, walnuts, and barbecue sauce.
8. Stir until every ingredient has been coated with the sauce.

9. Arrange the lentil mixture on a platter, and then top it with the coated chicken.
10. Serve immediately.

Yield: 2 to 3 servings

Tip: In case you do not have a rice cooker, you can use a small saucepan instead. Just bring it to a boil and then cover it. Simmer it for 10 to 15 minutes, or until most of the liquid has been absorbed, and the lentils are almost cooked through. At this point, add the asparagus and cook until the asparagus has become tender.

Miso Beef Noodle Soup

Ingredients:

- 1/2 lb. flank steak, thinly sliced
- 2 carrots, peeled and thinly sliced
- 4 scallions, chopped
- 4 garlic cloves, minced
- 1/2 lb. shiitake mushrooms, stems removed and thinly sliced
- 1/4 cup cilantro, chopped
- 2 tbsp. mellow white miso paste
- 6 oz. udon or ramen noodles, cooked according to packaging instructions
- 2 cups of low-sodium beef broth
- 2 cups of packed baby spinach leaves
- 2 cups of water
- 1 tbsp. of canola oil

Instructions:

1. Place flank steak on a flat surface or plate.
2. Rub miso paste, garlic, and cilantro on both sides of the steak. Set aside.
3. Heat a large stockpot using the high setting. Add canola oil.
4. Place steak inside the pot.
5. Cook for 2 to 3 minutes or until the meat has turned brown on the outside.

6. Transfer the steak to a plate.
7. Add carrots, mushrooms, and scallions to the pot.
8. Cook while stirring often for 3 to 4 minutes or until mushrooms have begun to soften.
9. Add beef broth and water to the pot.
10. Reduce heat from high to low.
11. Add noodles and cover.
12. Cook while stirring occasionally for 2 to 3 minutes or until noodles are cooked through.
13. Add spinach.
14. Return the meat to the pot once the spinach leaves have wilted.
15. Transfer into serving bowls.
16. Serve immediately.

Yield: 3 to 4 servings

Conclusion

Congratulations on making it to the end of this metabolic diet guide! We hope our insights have given you a better understanding of weight gain, its symptoms, and how the metabolic diet guide can help you achieve your health and wellness goals.

Weight gain is a complex issue that can have a significant impact on your physical and mental well-being. The good news is that by taking proactive steps toward improving your metabolic health, you can reduce your risk of chronic diseases and improve your overall quality of life.

The metabolic diet guide is an effective tool to help you achieve sustainable weight loss and long-term health benefits. By incorporating principles such as balanced macronutrient intake, high protein foods, low glycemic index foods, and frequent small meals, you can rev up your metabolism and promote fat burning.

While many diets promise quick results, the metabolic diet guide is designed to be a lifestyle change that leads to long-term success. It's important to work with a healthcare professional or registered dietitian to ensure that you are meeting your nutritional needs while adhering to the principles of the metabolic diet guide.

Incorporating healthy, whole foods, staying hydrated, getting regular exercise, and practicing stress management techniques can all help you achieve your weight loss and health goals. With consistent effort and commitment, you can overcome weight gain and achieve a healthier, happier life.

Remember, no journey towards better health is without its challenges, setbacks, or temptations. However, by adopting a positive mindset, prioritizing self-care, and seeking support from loved ones and professionals, you can stay motivated and progress toward your goals.

In conclusion, weight gain is a manageable condition, and the metabolic diet guide offers an effective tool to help you achieve sustainable weight loss and long-term health benefits. Remember to take it one step at a time, seek support from healthcare professionals, and prioritize your overall well-being. When you commit to your health, the possibilities are endless. So, take action today and start your journey towards a healthier, happier life!

References and Helpful Links

About overweight and obesity (For teens)—Nemours kidshealth. (n.d.). Retrieved May 6, 2023, from https://kidshealth.org/en/teens/obesity-overweight.html.

Endorphins: What they are and how to boost them. (n.d.). Cleveland Clinic. Retrieved May 6, 2023, from https://my.clevelandclinic.org/health/body/23040-endorphins.

How protein can help you lose weight naturally. (2017, May 29). Healthline. https://www.healthline.com/nutrition/how-protein-can-help-you-lose-weight.

Sleep loss boosts hunger and high-calorie food choices | University of Chicago News. (2016, March 1). https://news.uchicago.edu/story/sleep-loss-boosts-hunger-and-high-calorie-food-choices.

Weight loss benefits for arthritis | arthritis foundation. (n.d.). Retrieved May 6, 2023, from https://www.arthritis.org/health-wellness/healthy-living/nutrition/weight-loss/weight-loss-benefits-for-arthritis.

Weight loss plateau: Why they happen and what to do. (2019, September 23). https://www.medicalnewstoday.com/articles/326415.